Ketogenic Diet

The Secret High-Fat Diet

Contents

Introduction

Much has been made of all sorts of quick-weight loss, and fad diets, all delivering the promise of a slimmer figure, glowing good looks, and good health forever and ever. Unfortunately, that is all that they deliver: PROMISES. The slimmer figure and good looks may last for a little while, but the good health facet may not even be achieved even if the weight loss objectives are met.

The problem with these diets is that they were only designed for short-term weight loss, and if we really want to talk about diets, we know that over 97% of dieters get back the pounds that they have lost, and in many cases, actually gain more than what they originally weighed in the first place!

That is for only one diet - people spend a lot of their time going on diets, and the results are hardly successful. In a 2007 study, it was learned that women spend, on the average, 31 years of their lives going on a diet; just exceeding the number of years that men spend, 28.

Another problem with diets is that they usually require a drastic change in the eating patterns. Many require a dramatic drop in caloric intake. Some diets require that people eat tasteless and unappealing foods, making them want to end their diets quickly, and they just revert to their old eating patterns.

The diet that I will lead you through, Ketogenic Diet, is not a fad diet, and its underlying principles have been around for decades. In fact, Ketogenic Diet has not only been a sure-fire approach to weight loss. It has been used to treat certain health conditions, and help others avoid various illnesses.

Our Ketogenic Diet journey will be an educational one on nutrition and diet, and ultimately, a ticket to a better body, and glowing health. This book is divided into two parts, with Part I (Chapters 1 to 4) providing a background on the nutrition and health aspects of any diet. In Chapter 1, we will look at the roles of fat, carbohydrates, and protein in our nutrition, including a history of how humans have regressed to increasing rates of obesity, heart disease, and metabolic problems.

In Chapter 2, we look at how the human body uses the foods that we eat, and convert them into energy and tissue. Chapter 3 describes the body's descent into obesity, including the role of carbohydrates in this sometimes deadly process. We will talk about the various ailments and diseases that arise from a nutrition program with faulty information and premises. In Chapter 4, we review the concept of ketogenesis in detail, including the mechanics of how and why ketones are produced.

Part II of the book (Chapters 5 to 8,) will discuss the how to's for starting on, and progressing with Ketogenic Diet. Chapter 5 will discuss the objectives of the diet, including the significance of ketosis, and provide dieting patterns and schedule to follow. Chapter 6 will detail what foods should be eaten in the diet, and what should be avoided.

Chapter 7 will discuss the basic pointers on how to succeed on the diet. On the flipside, the chapter will also point out what traps to avoid. Chapter 8 gets down to the real world of Ketogenic Diet: Actual recipes that will provide you with a week's worth of meals, snacks, and even desserts, with an emphasis on getting you on a tasty and flavorful track to a healthier life style.

Ketogenic Diet has had a growing number of devotees and fans because of the documented success of millions who have tried it. There are also a growing number of health professionals, including M.D.'s and dieticians who have gone public in promoting the benefits of Ketogenic Diet.

A growing number of nutritionists have also began to assail the prescribed "balanced" diets that continue to be endorsed by official, national and international medical associations and even, governments. Many Ketogenic Diet devotees now dismiss these official pronouncements as downright wrong, and even, dangerous.

In this book, we will set the record straight on dietary fat and more precisely, its role in the human health and well-being.

We will see that dietary fat deserves to be elevated as THE food nutrient of choice, and should be consumed in at least equal quantities, as carbohydrates and proteins. Fat is not only recommended, but required, as a component of healthy eating and well-being, to help assure you a life of optimal vitality and health!

PART I – BACKGROUND INFORMATION

Chapter 1. The False Promises of Carbohydrates

Mankind's original fuel

All engines need fuel and energy, and human beings, as the most complicated naturally-occurring engine in existence, is no exception. While we put gasoline as fuel in cars, as human beings, we also need to have our own fuel, and this fuel is food. More precisely, food that will be needed in relatively large amounts, consumed consistently and regularly.

Our fuel, food, is comprised of three basic macronutrients: carbohydrates, fat and protein. Everything we eat as fuel for storage and energy comes from these three macronutrients. The human body needs these to function properly. How has the consumption of macronutrients changed over the last 10,000 years or so and what has brought us to this world of dieting and more correctly, failures in dieting?

Gog

Let me introduce you to "Gog," a typical ancestor from our prehistoric days, from about 10,000 years ago, give or take a few hundred years. Gog was a male member of the most advanced and latest version of homo sapien, of which we eventually became the proud descendants. In that stage of human history, Gog was part of that group called the "hunter-gatherers," who sourced their food from animals that they hunted and killed, and from fruits or berries that they happened to come across in their hunting adventures.

Gog and other co-inhabitants of the planet at that time subsisted on a diet that consisted mostly of animal fats, protein, and fibrous berries and fruits. Their Vitamin D source was principally the sun, and they had little use for plant carbohydrates, from whose chlorophyll content merely transfers the sun's Vitamin D nutrients.

Gog stayed out in the sun for most of the day, and the sun provided his "D". Vitamin D was, and continues to be important to sustain the human's bodily functions, but it is clear that fat was to be the human's primary source of fuel.

It is important to note that even today; certain tribes and cultures subsist on essentially high-fat diets and thrive with robust health. The Maasai group in Africa and Eskimos are modern day cultures that are known for the very small part that carbohydrates play in their diet. These groups are sustained by high fat diets in particularly unforgiving weather conditions. Apparently, their low-carbohydrate lifestyles have turned their metabolisms around to fat burners, rather than glucose burners.

This low-carbohydrate situation seemed to be the way that nature designed humans and their fuel needs: Man got their energy from fat, and fat was their fuel. For millions of years, the genius of nature, or even the genius of a Creator deemed that fat would be man's primary source of energy.

Was this simple diet enough for Gog's sustenance and health? For this, we can look at the archaeological record. On the next page, we present a table that shows life expectancy from the year 9,000 B.C., when agriculture, tilling the soil for carbohydrate foods, is generally is known to have started.

TABLE 1.

Life Expectancy of Our "Lithic Ancestors"

Period of Time	Ave. height -male	Ave. height - female	Life expectancy - Male	Life expectancy - Female
30,000 to 9,000 B.C. (Meat and fat is about 2/3 of the diet)	177.1 (5'9.7)	166.5 (5'5.6)	35.4	30.0
9,000 to 7,000 B.C. (Some agriculture already started – Meat and fat is now less than	172.5 (5'7.9)	159.7 (5'2.9)	33.5	31.3

1/3 of the diet)				
7,000 to 5,000 B.C. (Agriculture spreads widely in the Early Neolithic age – Meat is now 30% of the diet)	169.6 (5'6.8)	155.5 (5'1.2)	33.6	29.8
5,000 to 3,000 B.C. ("Late Neolithic," i.e., the transition	161.3 (5'3.5)	154.3 (5'0.7)	33.1	29.2

towards full blown agriculture is mostly complete)				
3,000 to 2,000 B.C. (Early Bronze Era)	166.3 (5'5.4)	152.9 (5'0.2)	33.6	29.4

The above table shows that when humanity began the agricultural stage, life expectancy actually decreased! The decrease should actually have been bigger if we factor in the increased physical security that our ancestors had because of agriculture: enclosed communities and better defensive mechanisms and positions against predatory animals. In fact, deaths from predators on the general population would be reduced to almost zero, with fatalities coming from predators only occurring with the armed male hordes that elected to hunt for animals.

Gog consumed just what his body required, and most of what he consumed was fat from whatever animals he hunted down. The fat he consumed was burned immediately and quickly, not because of physical activity per se, but because the human body, unlike a car, consumes and uses up energy even while he is in a state of rest and even sleep.

From Chapter 2, we will learn that the carbohydrates he consumed were immediately expended for quick bursts of energy. Gog therefore used his nutrients efficiently and effectively, not requiring much fat to be manufactured or stored. This is something we will come back to later in Chapter 4, when we talk about the mechanics of the diet.

"Post" Gog

The archaeological record also shows that as agriculture began to produce more food, agricultural plant products began to play a bigger role in the human diet. When human beings retreated into safer and cozier settlements, there was less of a need to go out and secure animal foods for food. Also note from the table, that males had higher life expectancies than females, even when their lives appeared to be in more mortal danger, being the hunters.

Humans, especially the male hunters, often turned into prey for the animals of the day. Despite this, males still had higher life expectancies because they presumably ate more of the fat that they hunted, possible consuming much of their meat immediately after securing them, and even before distributing them to their waiting families.

In a couple of thousand years more, meat, and especially fat, would continue to take a backseat to processed carbohydrates. Agriculture would become more efficient, and humans would not only produce more of carbohydrate foods, especially in the form of wheat and rice, they could store these foods longer!

For example, wheat and rice could be pounded down to flour, and stored in silos and bins over long periods of time. Because they could be stored longer, they became a much cheaper and more available source of sustenance and nutrition. After all, why risk lives hunting for food when it could be retrieved in a matter of minutes from a storage bin?

Health problems increase

As time marched on, life expectancies would increase as humankind learned more about medicines, while infant mortality rates would plummet. By the Middle Ages, average life expectancies would approach 50 years or so, but other mortal problems would surface: obesity, heart disease, and metabolic issues. Increased carbohydrate intake would totally throw human metabolic processes into crisis.

Before we get into the science and chemistry of food, we can historically trace these problems to one thing: Humans stopped eating naturally, and more importantly, reduced their intake of fat. Millions of years of eating unprocessed foods and fat were in the millennial blink of an eye, overturned, and the human body was shocked, and not pleasantly, to the new nutritional realities. Natural and fat was out, processed and carbohydrates were in. So-called blood diseases, and all sorts of unidentified diseases, presumably cancer and diabetes, began to spread.

Modern Man Doubles Down on the Carbohydrate Problem

From the middle ages to well into the 20th century, humankind saw an increasing, if not alarming incidence of heart disease and symptoms reflecting diabetes. Archaeologists, who have studied heart disease not surprisingly, found that heart disease was extremely rare in pre-industrial societies. After the so-called "Industrial Revolution," which gave witness to large-scale mechanization, heart and metabolic diseases shot up, and people were all of a sudden getting sick in newer ways. Heart attacks and symptoms attributable to strokes suddenly took hold.

Modern conventional wisdom, however, attributed this rise in diseases to the sedentary lifestyle that the advances in technology, especially the invention of machines, brought. The thinking was people were getting fatter and sicker, not because of food, but because people were doing less manual labor than from thousands of years ago. "Experts" assumed that fat deposits formed because people didn't exercise or were sitting, or lying around more.

What they missed or ignored was how human diet was drastically transformed when agriculture took over the human food supply. Modern technology not only made people move around less, it also helped mass produce agricultural products at a faster and cheaper pace.

After wheat and rice were produced in huge, mass proportions, sugar production finally became widespread in the 1700's, and made food, especially, carbohydrates, taste much better. Well into the 1900's, foods high in processed carbohydrate content, such as pizza, French fries, candies, and processed dairy foods gained shot up in popularity.

Moreover, processed carbohydrates became popular because of the short amount of time required to prepare, and with the advent of the microwave oven, cook them. Fast food became a symbol of modern society, and these foods are mostly all about carbohydrates in most of its forms: popcorn, potato chips, and candy bars being the most widespread and popular.

The growth of carbohydrates was largely ignored as a cause of increased heart disease. Because the true villain for human health was being overlooked, a boogeyman had to be found or invented – dietary fat.

Fat gets a bad rap

Sometime in the 1990s, fat was beginning to get demonized. It quickly became the dirty word of the nutrition industry and it was fashionable to shun as a deadly health hazard. Doctors derided it as a scourge to physical well-being, and consumers followed the medical herd, making fat as the primary source of a bunch of physical ailments, most of them revolving around the heart. High "bad" cholesterol, weight gain, artery disease, you name it – all of these were blamed on fat.

The curious thing about the demonization of fat was that there wasn't (and there still isn't) adequate scientific proof to back up these claims of nutritional Armageddon arising from fat.

Despite what science failed to prove, everyone jumped on the low-fat bandwagon, consuming mass quantities of food that, while indeed lacking fat, were instead, loaded with carbohydrates, especially sugar. The results of this "diet revolution" were that the average American got more obese, and the rate of increase of heart problems hastened.

According to U.S. Department of Health and Human Services statistics, by 2001, roughly a third of the American population was already overweight. This, of course, came with the increase in the incidence of heart disease and diabetes also soared.

The result of this "conventional wisdom" was that fresh whole foods such as meat, eggs, and their fatty components—the foods our ancestors ate for centuries—were being quickly replaced with low-fat "Frankenfoods" such as margarine, low-fat snack cookies, and skim milk. These foods were not only full of sugar and carbohydrates; some were also loaded with artificial ingredients. When these substances are consumed regularly, over time, the human body reacts by gaining weight, showing symptoms of fatigue and brain fog, and succumbing to chronic conditions.

Although scientific research produced findings to the contrary, fat—especially saturated fat—had developed a lasting reputation for being bad. Although the low-fat diet craze eventually dwindled, the damage was done. Fat was shunned and carbohydrates were placed on the nutritional pedestal.

In fact, government authorities began to promote, and still promote, the consumption of mostly carbohydrates, for their recommended dietary combinations. The National Institutes of Health, for example, continue to suggest that 70% of a diet should be comprised of carbohydrates in various forms. Subsequently, in the "Dietary Guidelines for America, 2015-2020," issued by the U.S. Department of Agriculture, dietary fats are merely mentioned almost as a footnote as oils.

The USDA also says that food oils (not fat) are limited to fat in liquid form, while naming vegetable cooking oils as the only source of fat nutrients that should be available for human consumption. There is no mention of the animal fat that our ancestors like Gog consumed, which was actually the main source of his energy fuel. The USDA caps their dismissal of fat by allowing very limited consumption levels of animal fat for the "ideal" diet.

To disseminate this fat-starved diet, the USDA pictorialized their concept of an ideal diet with the "My Plate" diagram, which portrays this dismissal of animal fat from the daily diet. The "Plate" emphasizes vegetables, fruits, grains, and protein, and assigns dairy as a supplemental item on the plate diagram. This diagram suggests that at least sixty percent of a person's recommended calorie intake should be comprised of foods from carbohydrates, which make up grains, vegetables, and fruits.

Fats from non-aquatic animals as beef, pork, and lamb, have been excluded in the nutritional conversation, with the "Plate" admonishing everyone to shun the so-called "trans-fat". Government agencies' objective is to limit the consumption of red meat, cheese, and processed meats.

The USDA recommended "Plate" is depicted as follows:

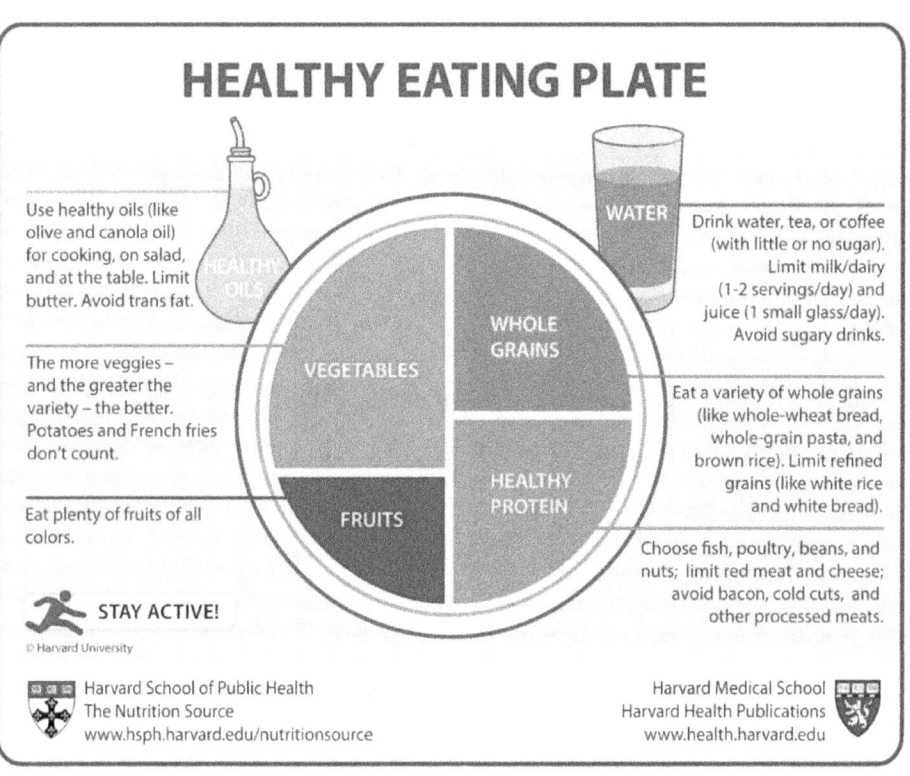

HEALTHY EATING PLATE

Use healthy oils (like olive and canola oil) for cooking, on salad, and at the table. Limit butter. Avoid trans fat.

The more veggies – and the greater the variety – the better. Potatoes and French fries don't count.

Eat plenty of fruits of all colors.

STAY ACTIVE!

© Harvard University

WATER
Drink water, tea, or coffee (with little or no sugar). Limit milk/dairy (1-2 servings/day) and juice (1 small glass/day). Avoid sugary drinks.

Eat a variety of whole grains (like whole-wheat bread, whole-grain pasta, and brown rice). Limit refined grains (like white rice and white bread).

Choose fish, poultry, beans, and nuts; limit red meat and cheese; avoid bacon, cold cuts, and other processed meats.

HEALTHY OILS · VEGETABLES · WHOLE GRAINS · FRUITS · HEALTHY PROTEIN

Harvard School of Public Health
The Nutrition Source
www.hsph.harvard.edu/nutritionsource

Harvard Medical School
Harvard Health Publications
www.health.harvard.edu

Source: U.S. Department of Agriculture

Nevertheless, many current scientific studies have not only repudiated the omission of animal fats from the diet, but have argued that fat from animals is not just a necessary component of the human diet, but should be accepted as the largest part of human nutrition. This is especially true when someone is endeavoring to lose weight, and eventually, get healthier.

The USDA, the National Institutes of Health, the World Health Organization, our grandparents, physicians, and even our gym instructors have been telling us what to eat. Now after we have followed their recommendations, and of course, our own palate, we consume the food and enjoy them. Sometimes, we don't really enjoy these, but just follow the herd to appear to stay modern and in touch. Regardless of what we eat, certain things happen in our body to convert all those goodies into energy.

Chapter 2. The Chemistry of Eating

In Chapter 1, we mentioned that food is the fuel that provides human beings with energy. The three macronutrients, carbohydrates, protein, and of course, fat are the fuels that power our bodies 24/7, day in and day out, whether we are moving around, resting, or even sleeping. In this chapter, we see the role of the macronutrients in the sustenance of our bodies, and how food is converted into fuel and other substances in our body.

Our bodies are highly intelligent, and yet, "needy" machines.

They know exactly what they want, and more importantly, what they need. The most unconscious of these needs, and yet probably the most important, is the need for fuel to provide our bodies with energy. Without these energy sources, our cells would starve to death.

You see all these shows and movies about people stranded in islands, forests, and deserts without food? Those are the consequences when your conscious minds and bodies cannot get the fuel necessary to function, and endure.

The first step, the easy and conscious part; chewing and swallowing, puts food into our bodies. The next, more important, however subconscious step; happens inside our body -- to break down this food for absorption, and conversion into energy. This process is called metabolism.

<u>Eating up</u>

Metabolism describes the chemical reactions that take place to maintain the dynamic state of our bodies and their constituent cells. Metabolism has two subordinate bodily functions to process the food/fuel, which we can conveniently divide into the following:

Catabolism – This refers to the breakdown of the molecules that we ingest. The macronutrients are broken down in substances and molecules that can be usable for the body to convert into fuel and energy.

Anabolism - This refers to the amalgamation of all compounds needed by the human body. Basically, in this stage, the body takes what has been broken down by catabolism, and processes the molecules to convert them to energy.

When we ingest the foods that contain the macronutrients of carbohydrates, fat, and proteins, our bodies immediately begin to work on the foods that we take in. The last conscious effort we have in this process is the swallowing of the foods that we have either chewed or drunk. When the mass of chewed food and/or liquids have passed our throat, and heads down our esophagus, the rest of body takes over beyond our conscious control. What happens to these foods?

In order to make sure that it always has access to energy; our body has several metabolic pathways it can use to convert the food that we eat into useable energy, and energy that we can store. We will summarize what these metabolic pathways are all about in the rest of this chapter.

For human beings, the default metabolic pathway is one that uses the glucose from carbohydrates as fuel. As long as you provide your body with carbohydrates, it will use them as energy, and storing excess macronutrients as fat in the process. When you deny your body of carbohydrates, it has to turn somewhere else to get the energy it needs to live. For millions of years up to about 9,000 years ago, the human body turned to mostly, stored and dietary fat.

Anabolism– fed and fasting states

In the metabolic process, a distinction also has to be made between the "fed" and the "fasting" state when the nutrients are being broken down during the anabolic stage. The fed state occurs about 4 hours after eating a meal or snack. This is the time when the body begins to absorb the digested nutrients. Some of these nutrients, especially carbohydrate-based ones, are used to meet immediate energy needs, while converting the extra nutrients to energy stored products.

In the "fasting state," which occurs 4 or more hours after eating, the body uses fat as its main source of energy. How fat or thin we are, depends on how much of fat stores are used, and of course, how those stores are built.

Let us now discuss these blessed little fuel sources.

Carbohydrates

These are probably the tastiest of all foods, the "lightest" on the mouth and the palate, the easiest to swallow, and from an economic standpoint, the cheapest. Rice and wheat for example, can be expanded to 2 or 3 times their original uncooked mass, then laced and mixed with all manner of sugars, creams, flavors, and texturized ingredients to provide the tastiest satisfaction from the lips to the tongue.

After we ingest carbohydrates, these are immediately broken down, by the introduction of various enzymes, into glucose, which is basically blood sugar. Some of the glucose is burned for instant energy, but usually, there is excess glucose left in the blood stream to trigger the body to try to regulate these increases in glucose.

Glucose is the body's favorite source of energy on demand, and is the fuel of choice for athletes, bodybuilders, and gym rats. This is why we have "sugar boosts" after consuming an energy bar or cookie, after a workout or an athletic exercise. The metabolic process that glucose undergoes is called "glycolysis," where the glucose is converted to mostly glycogen.

In the human body's infinite wisdom, it knows that too much glucose can be a problem (which we will see in a while.) To regulate the level of blood sugar, the body lets the pancreas release insulin, a regulating hormone. From this we can see that nature has considered carbohydrates to be inherently bad for the human body, otherwise, why limit it?

Indeed, nature has planted an organ in our body, the pancreas, to produce a singular hormone, insulin, to prevent the body from taking on too much blood sugar. We will visit insulin again in the next chapter when we talk about the effects of sugar and fat on the body.

Proteins

Proteins are responsible for creating the "building blocks" of our body tissues. The most common forms are lean meats and certain legumes. The foods containing protein provide more of a "chewing" sensation before being swallowed, provide the most "filling" sensation, and are more expensive per ounce, than carbohydrates.

Proteins are broken down into amino acids, and used by body cells to form either new proteins or to mixed up in some kind of amino acid "pool". This pool serves like a cache for the molecules, creating some sort of reservoir. Amino acids comprise a significant percentage of our body mass. A big percentage of our cells, tissues, and muscles are also comprised of amino acids.

Amino acids, therefore, perform a bunch of key body functions. One of the most paramount is giving our cells their form and structure. The metabolic process that protein undergoes is called "transamination," where the amino acids we eat are converted to glycogen or other protein compounds.

Aside from forming body tissues, amino acids play an important part in the storage and transport of essential nutrients. They have significant influence over the functions of arteries, glands, organs, and connective tissues, such as tendons. They also are indispensable for repairing tissues, and healing wounds, most especially in the skin, hair, bones, and muscles. Proteins also play an important role in the elimination of various waste deposits arising from metabolism.

Just as ingesting too much of carbohydrates is an issue, the body will need to "dispose" of "extra" amino acids produced over and above the body's requirements. The excess amino acids are transformed by enzymes in the liver into urea and keto acids. These keto acids can then be utilized as extra sources of energy, and via different anabolic processes, are transformed into glucose, or stored in the muscles as fat. Urine and sweat takes care of eliminating urea from the body.

Fat

Fat can be yummy, and can be gross at the same time, but fat is the king of human body fuels; nature having decreed it as the best source of energy. Fat from foods usually is ingested as part of other food items. For example, one can eat the fatty part of steaks, the skin of chickens, and the fat from fish, and egg yolks. Pure fat can be taken in limited forms: of such foods as whole milk and fried eggs.

When fats are eaten, they are converted into fatty acids and glycerol. They are digested in the person's small intestine.

They are then turned into lipoproteins for different essential functions (we will talk about bad and good cholesterol, LDL and HDL in the next chapter).

Getting energy from carbohydrates, proteins, and fat

When you eat, the nutrient molecules are absorbed in the intestine and into the bloodstream. In the fasting state, the cells will soon be taking up these nutrients and chemically burn them to liberate energy. The most common chemical fuel is the sugar glucose. Other molecules, such as fats or proteins, can also supply energy, but they usually have to first be converted to glucose or some intermediate that can be used in glucose metabolism.

This is where the energy superstar, adenosine triphosphate, or ATP, comes in. After all the three macronutrients are metabolized, ATP, a critical element in human metabolism, is produced when the body burns the sugars together with other nutrients. Mitochondria in the cells convert the food that we eat into ATP, which is a comparatively smaller molecule which functions as "energy intermediate" when we metabolize food.

ATP is often referred to as "chemical currency" as the body uses it as a direct energy source. The body produces ATP when it burns up various nutrients and sugars, while our cells ingest ATP when engaging in actions such as producing movement, and on an atomic scale, building larger molecules. Our cells then chemically process ATP, resulting in the release of energy, in order for the human body to engage in various activities.

In essence, our body cells take out the chemical energy from different nutrient molecules such as proteins and carbohydrates, and then utilize this chemical energy to produce ATP. How do we go from glucose to ATP? This is achieved through the process of "oxidation".

For example, glucose, the molecule that came from our consumption of carbohydrates, including many dietary sugars and starch, are broken down to make waste products like water and carbon dioxide. But our cells will utilize the energy freed up from breaking down a single glucose molecule, and produce about thirty ATP molecules.

As soon as a cell has produced ATP, it will now utilize the ATP to meet any of its energy requirements. Cells require energy in order to produce large molecules, such as hormones, for example. Muscle cells also make ATP to generate movement. As a cell produces a large molecule, ATP molecules are broken down. The cell utilizes this energy to produce original bonds among smaller molecules resulting in the production of a bigger one, and the process goes on.

All these processes occur amazingly without our conscious effort or thinking. Our bodies are amazing machines that do all these processes automatically. If we take in the right foods in the right amounts, there shouldn't be any problems. However, since the age of agriculture dawned on humanity 9,000 years ago or so, our bodies have unfortunately, not been so lucky.

Chapter 3. How We Get Fat and Sickness From Food

We now have an idea of how the body processes the macronutrients. Let us pay attention to the negative side of eating, and what happens when we take in too much of the "wrong" types of food into our bodies, especially carbohydrates. In the previous chapter, we mentioned that our bodies were "intelligent" in the singular sense that it tells us when we need fuel, and signals our bodies to take in food whenever our energy sources are getting low.

On the flipside, however, our bodies cannot be "smart enough" to totally withstand bad nutrition, which is eating foods that were not originally designed for our consumption. Despite our bodies' best "efforts," we become obese and sick, and there is very little that it can do from a self-defense standpoint to fight this. In nutrition, the worst thing that can happen to the human body, aside from not being fed enough, is being fed too much, and worse, being fed too much of the wrong foods.

The sugar curse

It may seem that carbohydrates, especially sugars, will be demonized in this, and other books, as the benefits of low-carb, high-fat diets continue to portray as the correct way towards proper weight loss and good health. Actually, as we have seen in the previous chapter, sugar by itself, is not the problem. In fact, we talked about the importance of glucose, and how even proteins and fats are broken down to make sugar in the body.

Glucose is absolutely essential to life, and our metabolism cannot function properly without it. Each cell in our body is able to utilize glucose as energy. Even when we cannot obtain glucose from our diet directly, we can get what we need from fats and proteins. In fact, we have a constant supply of it in our bloodstream. But it can also create severe problems.

<u>Too much sugar</u>

We have discussed how processed carbohydrates, because of their lower price, accessibility, and taste, have become the most consumed macronutrient. The fact that they are also the "lightest" on the mouth and the palate, added to carbohydrates' promotion as the preferred macronutrient, it has practically ensured that human beings will eat them more than any other food.

But sugary and carbohydrate-packed foods are also the most easily converted and metabolized macronutrient. They pass through the digestive tract the fastest, and these factors combined ensure that too much of carbohydrates can be eaten, especially if the habit is picked up when we are young. The bottom line is that anytime we fill our bodies with more than the needed fuel levels, the storage capacity of our liver for sugar is exceeded, and sometimes, greatly.

The liver can store up to only around 5% of its mass as glycogen, which has been converted from excess glucose. When the liver is packed at close to full capacity, the excess sugars are transformed by the liver into more fatty acids.

Worse, these fatty acids go back into the bloodstream, and is distributed throughout our bodies and stored as fat! These fats are stored away where our bodies are designed to store these as adipose fat cells. These areas include, but not limited to, the popular regions of the butt, breasts and hips for women, and the stomach for men. These fatty cells can also imbed themselves in the arteries, causing arteries to deteriorate and being clogged with fat and debris from extra fat.

As a disastrous reverse bonus, as soon as these areas become full with fatty tissues and adipose cells, they will start to leak over into our vital organs – these include the kidneys, liver, and heart. The presence of fat will impair and impede the organ's ability to perform, raise blood pressure, lower metabolic rates, cause a feeling of constant tiredness, and expose the body to illness and sickness as our immune system is weakened.

The body pushes excess glucose into the cells to be made into ATP, or stored as glycogen which are converted into fat droplets called triglycerides in the fat cells, or adipose tissue. "New fat" has just been created.

The wrong sugars

Compounding the "too much" sugar problem is that we may not only be eating too much of carbohydrates, but humans, more than ever, are consuming the wrong carbohydrates. "Gog" and our prehistoric ancestors filled their bellies with natural berries, natural wild fruit, and natural fibers. The operative was natural, and Gog only ate foods that nature provided.

Today, however, there are a vast multitude of foods that contain sugars that nature did not intend us to ingest. Many foods, especially desserts, have sugar (sucrose) and high fructose corn syrup. These are sweetening agents that help enhance the taste of many foods and drinks – practically all non-diet sodas and ice creams contain them.

These are very different from natural sugars that contain glucose, which is an essential life giving nutrient, taken in the right quantities, but fructose is another matter. The molecule is not part of our normal metabolism and we do not produce it. A tiny fraction of cells in the human body can make use of it except liver cells. Since these cannot be properly assimilated into other cellular functions, they get turned to fat, and are eventually secreted into the blood.

Insulin and the Big D- Diabetes

We mentioned in the previous chapter that our bodies are intelligent enough to know that carbohydrates, and especially, processed sugars, are not good for the body, and it takes great pains to try to mitigate the effects of bad dietary habits. One of its best defense mechanisms is the pancreas, which secretes insulin to help mitigate the creation of too much blood sugars and fats, the results of which can be devastating, as we have seen above.

Insulin plays an indispensable role in the body. Its biggest role is its interaction with glucose to let our bodies utilize glucose properly as energy. The pancreas, the organ which produces insulin, excretes enough insulin and it acts as some sort of a "key" that allows the cells of the body to take in, and use glucose as energy.

Insulin assists in controlling blood glucose levels by alerting muscle cells, fat cells, and the liver to extract glucose from the blood. If our bodies have sufficient energy, insulin alerts our liver to process the incoming glucose, and store it as glycogen.

The glucose that insulin "pushes" in to the cells in the form of glycogen can then be transformed into ATP, or stored as fat as described earlier. This additional stored glycogen can then be utilized later on when the body needs more energy. When our bodies experience a disruption in the balance between fat production and the secretion of insulin, diabetes will occur.

Type1 Diabetes

This form of diabetes has also been called insulin-dependent diabetes or juvenile-onset diabetes, and accounts for less than 10 percent of all diabetes cases. Usually a genetic affliction, in this diabetes type, our body's immune system kills the cells that are responsible for releasing insulin, which in effect, stops insulin production.

Type 2 Diabetes

This is the type that Ketogenic Diet will most likely try to address. Type 2 diabetes is the most common form of diabetes (over 90% of diabetes cases), and is usually the result of a diet with very high in carbohydrates. The ones suffering the disease will manifest any symptom prior to diagnosis. Usually Type 2 diabetes is found during adulthood, although a few cases have been known to have been diagnosed in children.

In this affliction, our bodies cannot process insulin the right way. While the most common root cause is still debatable, there is a growing consensus that this is a "lifestyle" disease emanating from an overconsumption of carbohydrates. The bottom line is that the ability of the body to produce insulin has been overwhelmed by the amount of glucose produced. This condition is called, "insulin resistance," and eventually, the body will make less and less insulin, leading some to require insulin injections.

Since Type 2 Diabetes is a lifestyle disease, the way to deal with it is to change our lifestyles! This is best done by going on Ketogenic Diet, and getting the body into the ketosis state.

Chapter 4. Ketosis and Ketogenesis

The human body was designed to use fat for energy, and when mostly fat is used for energy, it does not store that fat, and the body becomes lean, as nature designed it. From Chapter 2, we found out that our bodies have several metabolic pathways it can use to convert the food that we eat into useable energy. The default metabolic pathway is one that uses the glucose from carbohydrates as fuel. As long as you provide your body with carbohydrates, it will use them as energy, storing fat in the process.

When you deny your body with carbohydrates, it has to turn somewhere else to get the energy it needs to live. If you starve your body of carbohydrates, therefore, the body will burn fat, and in the metabolic process, it will produce something called, "ketones." These are what may save your life!

Ketones are organic compounds that are made in the liver from fatty acids, and are generated from the breakdown of fats, especially when the body cannot "locate" any glucose to turn into energy. Ketones are formed almost as a defensive action by the body. When it "senses" that there is not enough sugar or glucose to provide for the body's energy needs, it immediately creates an alternative fuel source.

The Creation of Ketones and Ketosis

During times of fasting, or when we intentionally follow a low-carbohydrate diet, it turns to fat for energy. In simple terms, fat is taken to the liver where it is broken down into glycerol and fatty acids through a process called beta-oxidation. The fatty acid molecules are further broken down through a process called ketogenesis, and a specific ketone body called acetoacetate is formed.

If we continue on Ketogenic Diet, over time, our bodies will adapt to using ketones as fuel, and our muscles will convert the acetoacetate into beta-hydroxybutyrate or BHB. BHB is actually the preferred ketogenic source of energy for your brain, and acetone, most of which is expelled from the body as waste.

When dietary carbohydrates are suddenly taken away from the diet, more fatty acids are released from fat cells, which leads to more fat cells being burned up in our liver. This increase in the burning of fatty acids in the liver eventually causes ketone bodies to be produced, and induces ketosis, a new metabolic state.

Other hormones are likewise affected, and these help transfer the use of this new fuel, instead of carbohydrates, to body tissues. The majority of calories burned up by the human body will now come from this fat breakdown.

The glycerol created during the beta-oxidation process enters into a stage called gluconeogenesis. During gluconeogenesis, the body converts glycerol into glucose that your body can use for energy. Your body can also convert excess protein into glucose. Your body does need some glucose to function, but it doesn't need carbohydrates to get it. In other words, during this period, our body is beginning to now burn fat instead of converted sugar! Ketosis has set in, and hopefully for good!

<u>So is fat and ketosis bad?</u>
Ketogenic Diet has been at the forefront of a big diet "revolution" for the past few decades. Its popularity continues to increase, as new scientific evidence continues to surface, and proves that fat does not deserve the bad nutritional reputation it has received. Is fat bad?

The human body was designed to use fat for energy, no matter where it is produced. This results in a lean body, as nature originally designed it. How does a dieter on Ketogenic Diet get to ketosis? Getting to a state of ketosis means ingesting less than 50 grams of carbohydrates per day, and in the next Chapters we will find out how to count these carbohydrates, including the tools you need to measure carbohydrate intake.

Weight loss in Ketogenic Diet

Now that you understand how your body creates energy and how ketones are formed, you may be still wondering just how this translates into weight loss. Let's provide a quick review and summary.

When you eat a lot of carbohydrates, your body happily burns them for energy and stores any excess as glycogen in your liver, or as triglycerides in your fat cells. When we take carbohydrates out of the equation or reduce our intake of them drastically, our body depletes its glycogen stores in the liver and muscles and then turns to fat for energy.

When our bodies start to burn stored fat, our fat cells shrink and you begin to lose weight and become leaner. Smaller, leaner cells = smaller, leaner bodies!

Ketosis has sometimes been confused with ketoacidosis, which is a pre-existing condition present in some diabetic patients. It is a condition where there is not enough insulin produced in the body. Ketosis is not ketoacidosis, and vice-versa. Ketosis will not lead to ketoacidosis, and assuming you have no other medical conditions that may prevent you from going on Ketogenic Diet.

While many people try to dismiss Ketogenic Diet as a dangerous fad diet, it is well worth noting that the diet has many helpful, life-changing, and life-saving effects on our bodies and long-term health. Weight loss and looking great is sometimes viewed as merely side benefits by those who have stayed on the diet for an extended period of time.

There are other ways on how Ketogenic Diet can contribute to your well-being and long life. If you understand what amazing benefits are in store, it will be very easy to get convinced to stay on the diet. Described below are the foremost benefits of going on Ketogenic Diet.

Elimination of Type-II diabetes

We mentioned that Type-II diabetes is a lifestyle issue, and that it can be cured by a lifestyle change. For diabetes, the best lifestyle change is to get on Ketogenic Diet, and stop letting carbohydrates ruin your health. Many Type-II diabetes conditions are treatable before requiring the use of injected insulin.

Reduction of the symptoms of epilepsy

Ketogenic Diet is sometimes recommended to help control seizure symptoms in some patients afflicted with epilepsy. Ketogenic Diet is prescribed by a doctor and the patient undergoes careful monitoring under the watch of a professional dietitian.

Reduction in the symptoms of cancer

Cancer cells are very much not like our healthy cells. One way that they have known to be way different is that they have about ten times as many more insulin receptors on their surface as ordinary cells. The receptors allow the cells to feed on nutrients and glucose coming from the bloodstream at a very significant rate.

The more carbohydrates that are catabolized, the more glucose are produced which helps the cancer cells gorge for their "nutrition." If we are able to remove carbohydrates from our diets, we can possibly deny cancer cells from their energy source.

Reducing the incidence and severity of Parkinson's disease and Alzheimer's

Parkinson's disease is one of those "motor system" disorders where the onset happens between the ages of 50 and 65 years old. In the United States, about 1 percent of people in that age group are affected with it. In Parkinson's disease, the dopamine-producing cells in the brain are seemingly destroyed. The symptoms of Parkinson's disease include slowness of movement, trouble with balance, tremors, and shaking.

Near the terminal phase, the victim is usually on a wheelchair, or bed-ridden. These symptoms show up after up to 80 percent of the dopamine-producing cells in the brain are devastated. While it is not exactly clear on how Ketogenic Diet can alleviate the symptoms of Parkinson's disease, it is highly possible that ketones, which have an anti-inflammatory effect on the brain, may be able to fix impaired neurons.

The ketones may also possibly bypass the area in the brain that is damaged, and bring much-needed energy to other areas in the brain.

Reduction of symptoms of Mitochondrial Disorders

Mitochondria are organelles that are of significant numbers in most human cells. This is where the essential biochemical processes of energy production and respiration take place. Mitochondria are also considered as the energy centers of the human body. They convert the food that we eat to adenosine triphosphate, or ATP, as we have learned in Chapter 2.

When mitochondria become dysfunctional, the cells are denied of the energy they need. Because the brain, muscles, heart, nervous system, and eyes demand the most energy, their cells are often the most significantly affected with a mitochondrial disorder. Affecting these body parts cause learning and intellectual disabilities, muscle weakness, hearing and visual impairment, respiratory disorders, and even seizures. There is no cure for mitochondrial disorders, so their treatment focuses on alleviating its symptoms and improving the quality of life of the sufferer.

Proper diet is often the first stage of therapy for these disorders, and with seizures are a common symptom, a high-fat, Ketogenic Diet is often part of the treatment plan.

Reduction of symptoms of Lou Gehrig's or ALS Disease

ALS (Amyotrophic Lateral Sclerosis) is a progressive, neuro-degenerative ailment that assaults the nerve cells in the spinal cord and brain. ALS specifically affects the motor neurons, which are responsible for voluntary muscle movement. When motor neurons die, they are no longer able to send nerve signals to the muscle fibers leading to slurred speech, difficulty swallowing, muscle weakness, and almost instantly fatal breathing. At any rate, most of the muscles begin to waste away, and the person affected becomes weaker.

The exact cause of ALS is unknown, and there is no cure for the disease. Researchers believe that disruptions of the mitochondria in the brain and changes in a person's diet may help those with ALS, as well. Studies on mice and other animals show that those under Ketogenic Diet experienced a greater decrease in symptoms than those who weren't.

Improved Focus and Mental Clarity

For the brain, exposure to too much glucose can result in neurotoxicity or the exposure of the nervous system to toxic substances. Many mental issues, such as brain fog and problems with memory, are caused by this condition. In Ketogenic Diet, the reduction of the supply of glucose diminishes the levels of toxicity in the body as brain starts to use ketones as fuel. Possible results are the ability to think more clearly, better focus, and better memory recall.

Increased Energy

When the body breaks down fat instead of carbohydrates, more energy is produced for each ounce of fat used, leaving the Ketogenic dieter with a feeling of heightened alertness and increased energy.

Better heart and coronary health

When there are less fat cells flowing through the blood stream, that means that there is less strain on the heart and the arteries. This is a result of less plaque clogging up the bloodstream, and a better functioning circulatory system.

Lower "bad cholesterol" levels

Weight and fat loss are the objectives of an overwhelming majority of people going on Ketogenic Diet. Of course, the associated benefits of a slimmer body can also lead to a decrease in "bad" cholesterol levels, blood pressure, and just better heart health.

Breaking the myths surrounding high fat diets

It is useful to know what people, even health professionals, can say to scare people from Ketogenic Diet. There are many myths and misconceptions that have surrounded, and clouded ketosis and Ketogenic Diet.

Ketosis myths

Myth 1: Carbohydrates are an essential nutrient for good health.

Myth2: Eating a low-carbohydrate diet can lead to vitamin deficiencies, especially Vitamin C, which come from carbohydrate-rich sugary fruits and vegetables.

Myth 3: Ketogenic Diet causes your body to go into ketoacidosis, which is dangerous.

Myth 4: Your kidneys will sustain damage from high fat consumption.

Myth 5: A high-fat diet will lead to osteoporosis, because it will cause the body to excrete calcium.

Myth 6: Eating fat makes you fat.

Myth 7: Ketogenic Diet leaves out carbohydrates completely.

Myth 8: Cholesterol from animal fat causes heart diseases.

PART II – Ketogenic Diet

Chapter 5. Ketogenic Diet Basics

Before we get into the nitty-gritty of the diet, an important few words on how Ketogenic Diet is different from other low-carbohydrate diets on the market.

<u>Atkins Diet</u>

Atkins Diet was at the forefront of the low carbohydrate revolution and brought ketosis and ketogenesis into public awareness about fifty years ago. Atkins Diet allows for a moderate amount of protein in the menu. The allowable ratio is about 50-35-15 in terms of fat/protein/carbohydrate ratio. In Ketogenic Diet, the overwhelming amount of calories should come from fat, about 70%.

Atkins Diet also puts a lot of emphasis on the two week, "induction" phase, where the dieter will have to consume the required macronutrients. Atkins Diet promoters claim that a person can lose up to fifteen pounds on the first week of the diet.

Atkins Diet also allows the dieter to slowly reintroduce certain carbohydrates after the induction period. On Ketogenic Diet, the dieters need to be on a high fat diet for the rest of their lives.

Paleolithic Diet

Paleolithic Diet focuses on the foods supposedly eaten by our prehistoric ancestors, just like Ketogenic Diet, and also reduces the emphasis on carbohydrates. But Paleolithic Diet also allows for more significant portions of vegetables and certain fruits. Certain grains are allowed, and in fact recommended. Like Ketogenic Diet, Paleolithic Diet forbids tubers and sweet potatoes. The big difference between both diets is that high fat dairy products can be consumed on Ketogenic Diet, but is expressly disallowed on Paleolithic Diet.

Other diets that promote lower carbohydrate intake

Two other famous diets, Zone Diet and South Beach Diet, also recommend carbohydrate intake significantly lower than that of Ketogenic Diet. However, they allow for the consumption of a wider variety of carbohydrates. Ultimately, only Ketogenic Diet dictates that the significant majority of macronutrients consumed should be from fat.

The importance of macronutrients

Our body's overwhelming source of fuel is the food that we eat. Some of our energy comes from sunlight (Vitamin D), but 99% of our fuel comes from macronutrients in the food that we eat.

Ketogenic Diet's effectiveness depends almost wholly on what we eat and drink. There is no need for supplementation, such as vitamins when we go on Ketogenic Diet.

Think of the macronutrients as the gasoline that we put in our cars. Taking in the wrong macronutrients can be compared with putting contaminated fuel in your gas tank, or putting diesel fuel, for example, in a car that requires high-octane gasoline.

In Ketogenic Diet, the proper fuel is fat.

Getting on Ketogenic Diet

a. Prepare your household and cupboard for Ketogenic Diet

Going on a high-fat diet means a big change in lifestyle. If we are not living alone, and have to share our cupboards, refrigerators, and shopping budgets with other people, we need to properly announce that things will be changing drastically in the food storage department.

On Ketogenic Diet, carbohydrates are the big enemy, and we have to make sure that no "stealth carbs" manage to intrude our food space. Be organized, create lists, and shop carefully. We go into much greater detail on what we need to eat in the next chapter.

b. How many grams of protein, carbs and fats should be eaten in Ketogenic Diet?

In Chapter 1, we mentioned that most "authorities" recommend that about two thirds of calories should come from carbohydrates. This means that for a typical daily diet of 2,000 calories consumed, at least 1,300 calories of the total should be consumed in the form of carbohydrates. Additionally, around 500 calories should come from protein, and the remainder, should come from incidental, and trace quantities of fat.

Remember that these so called authorities do not even contemplate fat as being a food group, but only gives some token credit to fats as oils added to foods for taste and use in food preparation.

Ketogenic Diet turns this all around. Dietary fat should now make up about two-thirds of daily calorie consumption, allowing a maximum of ten percent to come from carbohydrates. Converting this to food weights, this means that under Ketogenic Diet, we should only consume daily between 30 and 50 grams of carbohydrates.

The more active a person is, however, a little more carbohydrates are added, maybe up to 100 grams, can be eaten. This is a concession to the fact that carbohydrates are useful for those that require short-term bursts of energy, such as those who go to a gym or exercise regularly and athletes.

For protein, the recommended quantity can be between 115 grams and 175 grams per day. The rest of the diet should be concentrated on fat. For a 2,000 calorie daily diet, we need to ingest at least 60%, or 1,200 calories of fat, 25%, or 500 calories from protein, and 15%, or 300 calories, from carbohydrates.

A note on protein which we have given very little attention to: Proteins are important in the creation, maintenance, and repair of muscle tissues. We want protein to rebuild our tissue, and not be an inefficient source of energy. In fact, excess proteins can turn into fat, the way carbohydrates are converted.

c. Recording and monitoring calorie and macronutrient intake

To ensure of the success of the diet, we need to carefully monitor how much of each macronutrient we are consuming daily, to ensure that the right proportion of calories are being consumed.

There are a multitude of carbohydrate/calorie counters that are available. The preeminent source is the suite of Atkins

Diet publications that pioneered the high-fat revolution. These need to be purchased in publication or app form.

A good source to look for apps is http://www.mydreamshape.com/carb-counter-apps/

Regardless of whether you record your progress in a written journal, or monitor yourself via computer, tablet, or phone, you need to strictly be in compliance with the percentages I have just mentioned. This monitoring is especially important in the first few weeks, when you are transitioning your body into the ketosis state.

Of course, you need to pay strict attention to the actual macronutrients you can (and should not!) consume when you are on the diet.

d. Signs That You Are in Ketosis

Signs that you're in ketosis may start appearing after only one week of following a true Ketogenic Diet. For some people, it can take longer—as much as three months. The amount of time it takes for you to start seeing signs that your body is burning fat for fuel largely depend on you as an individual. When signs do start to show, they are pretty similar across the board.

"Keto Flu"

"Keto flu" or "low-carb flu" commonly affects people in the first few days of starting Ketogenic Diet. Of course, Ketogenic Diet doesn't actually cause the flu, but the phenomenon is given the term because its symptoms closely resemble that of the flu. It would be more accurate to refer to this stage as a carbohydrate withdrawal, because that's really what it is.

When you take carbohydrates away, it causes altered hormonal states and electrolyte imbalances that are responsible for the associated symptoms. The basic symptoms include headache, nausea, upset stomach, sleepiness, fatigue, abdominal cramps, diarrhea, and lack of mental clarity, or what is commonly referred to as "brain fog."

Carbohydrate addiction is a real thing. Some research shows that carbohydrates activate certain stimuli in the brain that can be dependence-forming and cause addiction. Carbohydrate addicts have uncontrollable cravings for carbohydrates, and when they do eat them, they tend to binge. For a carbohydrate addict, the removal of carbohydrates can cause withdrawal symptoms, such as dizziness, irritability, and intense cravings.

The duration of the symptoms varies—it depends on you as an individual, but typically "keto flu" lasts anywhere from a couple of days to a week. In rare cases, it can last up to two weeks. Some of the symptoms of the "keto flu" are associated with dehydration, because in the beginning stages of ketosis you lose a lot of water weight.

With that lost fluid, you also lose electrolytes. You can replenish these electrolytes by drinking enhanced waters (but make sure they are not sweetened) and drinking lots of homemade bone broth. This may help lessen the severity of the symptoms.

Bad Breath

Unfortunately, bad breath is another early sign that you're in ketosis. When you're in ketosis, your body creates acetone as a waste product. Some of this acetone is released in your breath, giving it a fruity or ammonia-like quality. You can combat bad breath by chewing on fresh mint leaves and drinking plenty of water, since bad breath is also associated with dehydration.

Decreased Appetite and Nausea

As your body adapts to Ketogenic Diet, you may have a decreased appetite. This is because you're providing your body with plenty of fat and protein, which are both highly satiating, and not a lot of carbohydrates. The nausea associated with "keto flu" can also decrease your appetite. When you reach this stage, it's important that you eat even if you feel like you aren't hungry. You want to make sure your body is getting enough calories and nutrients, especially in this time of transition.

Increased Energy

When the fog begins to clear and your body starts to become keto-adapted, the uncomfortable symptoms you were feeling will dissipate and you'll begin to see the benefits of following Ketogenic Diet. One of the first beneficial signs many people experience is an increase in energy. When your body breaks down fat instead of carbohydrates, more energy is produced gram for gram, leaving you feeling alert and energized.

Other Possible Signs

Cold hands and feet

Increased urinary frequency

Difficulty sleeping

Metallic taste in the mouth

Dry mouth

Increased thirst

Chapter 6. What to Eat. And What Not to!

Shopping for the right foods is the first and most important step short of putting the right food in the mouth. For today's food shopper, fortunately, most food manufacturers are sensitive to the needs and requirements of people who go on special diets such as Ketogenic Diet. In labeling their foods, they have endeavored to be more accurate and responsive to people who need the proper information to go on their diets.

Regardless of whether foods are "allowed," the serious dieter will still have to make sure that they are staying well within the required macronutrient ratios (preferably 65% fat, 20% protein, and 15% carbohydrates). If measuring ratios are not possible during a given meal, the overriding principle is that the majority of the calories eaten daily should come from fat, and a very small percentage should be from carbohydrates.

Quality

The "quality" of your food matters, especially when it comes to fat and protein sources. Going back to the prehistoric time, our ancestors got healthy on unprocessed and unrefined food alone. It would be healthy and beneficial if a diet plan replicates that prehistoric food profile. A Ketogenic dieter should also try to purchase foods that have the following descriptions on the labels: organic, grass-fed, free-range, and/or pasture-raised.

Food with labels that say, "farm-raised" should be avoided as much as possible, because in all probability, whatever has been "raised" in those "farms" have been sprinkled with a healthy dose of chemicals and preservatives to improve yield and increase the animals' sizes.

Meats, poultry, and seafood

These are the staples of Ketogenic Diet, not vegetables, rice, or grains. They are the most plentiful, and in fact, appetizing components of the diet, and contains naturally-occurring fat. There are many foods in this group that most people can eat all they want every day. Foods included in this food group comprise all types of beef, chicken, turkey, duck, fish, lamb, pork, shrimp, crab, and lobster.

Of course, "exotic" varieties such as ostrich, goat, deer, and buffalo, are also allowed, if available. While bacon and sausage are excellent sources of protein and fat, care should be taken in eating processed meats, especially hotdogs and sausages. Many brands contain substantial quantities of carbohydrate fillers.

Remember that when eating meat, make sure to stay within your recommended protein grams for the day, since your body converts excess protein into glucose via glucogenesis, which can kick you out of the ketosis state.

In the following lists, we will show what the carbohydrate and fat contents are for a particular food item. Remember that these measurements are for uncooked and undressed food. Because Ketogenic Diet is ultimately a low-carbohydrate diet, we are listing the carbohydrate content of each food item. We will also list the number of calories for each item. Note that there may be many varieties of food types, especially in the meat items, because meat comes from various parts of the animal.

The list below is a fairly large general representation of foods that we generally eat. In the reference section of this book, I provide some resources for carbohydrate and calorie counting, in general.

a. Foods that are good for Ketogenic Diet

Animal Meats:

Beef/Veal – 3 oz. has 0 carbohydrates, and about 300 calories

Pork - 3 oz. has 0 carbohydrates, and about 200 calories

Lamb - 3 oz. has 0 carbohydrates, and about 175 calories

Goat - 3 oz. has 0 carbohydrates, and about 100 calories

Venison -3 oz. has 0 carbohydrates, and about 150 calories

Other wild game:

Keep in mind, the organic and grass-fed meat. Even if they are a little more expensive, they are the healthiest options, because there is a much lesser chance that they will contain growth hormones and preservatives. Game meat has generally less calories than regular pork and beef, and for the most part, has zero carbohydrates.

Processed meats:

While being basically comprised of the same meats that we have just listed that have zero carbohydrates, the curing and processing required to give them taste, sometimes necessitates the adding of carbohydrates.

Bacon – 3 oz. has less than 2 grams of carbohydrates, and about 450 calories

Bologna – 12-gram slice has about 1 gram of carbohydrates, and about 50 calories

Pork rinds - 3 oz. has 0 carbohydrates, and about 300 calories

Salami - 12-gram slice has about 1 gram of carbohydrates, and about 50 calories

Sausage (e.g., Bratwurst, Kielbasa, etc.) - 3 oz. has 2 grams of carbohydrates, and about 300 calories

Make sure that these yummy meats do not contain added sugars or excess preservatives.

Poultry:

You can be liberal with the skin and the fat portions. There is no need to skim them off anymore. Once again, organic and grass-fed cuts are the healthiest options. These include:

Chicken – 100 grams has 0 carbohydrates, and about 120 calories

Duck - 100 grams has 0 carbohydrates, and about 130 calories

Goose - 100 grams has 0 carbohydrates, and about 160 calories

Ostrich - 100 grams has 0 carbohydrates, and about 110 calories

Pigeon -100 grams has 0 carbohydrates, and about 200 calories

Quail - 100 grams has 0 carbohydrates, and about 150 calories

Turkey - 100 grams has 0 carbohydrates, and about 125 calories

Speaking of poultry, eggs, especially the yolk part, are highly recommended. Organic eggs or eggs from grass-fed chickens are preferred.

Fish – fatty varieties, especially:

Bass - 100 g has 0 carbohydrates, and about 150 calories

Halibut - 100 g has 0 carbohydrates, and about 110 calories

Mackerel - 100 g has 0 carbohydrates, and about 200 calories

Salmon - 100 g has 0 carbohydrates, and about 140 calories

Tuna - 100 g has 0 carbohydrates, and about 150 calories

Trout - 100 g has 0 carbohydrates, and about 150 calories

Peanut Butter – Check the labels to ensure that the variety is very low in carbohydrates, and have no sugar content. 2 tbsps. of such varieties have about 5 g of carbohydrates, and 200 calories.

Dairy:

Butter – 0 carbohydrates and 500 calories per 100 grams

Cheese – Make sure that you watch out for blends! They may have sugars and other dangerous chemicals and preservatives to make them look, and taste like real cheese. Most well-prepared cheese without any fillers 100 g has 1.5 g carbs, and about 400 calories

Plant products:

Asparagus, green – 1 cup has 5 g of carbohydrates and calories

Avocados - 1 cup has 20 g of carbohydrates and 300 calories

Bamboo shoots - 1 cup has 8 g of carbohydrates and 40 calories

Broccoli - 1 cup has 6 g of carbohydrates and 30 calories

Celery stalks - 1 cup has 4 g of carbohydrates and 15 calories

Coconuts – 1 cup has 12 g of carbohydrates and 300 calories

Green, leafy vegetables, such as bok choy, lettuce, Swiss card, radicchio, endives. These are non-starchy vegetables and typically 1 cup has about 5-10 g of carbohydrates and between 25-50 calories.

Kale - 1 cup has 5 g of carbohydrates and 30 calories

Kohlrabi - 1 cup has 8 g of carbohydrates and 40 calories

Radish - 1 cup has 2 g of carbohydrates and 15 calories

Broth, especially self-made bone broth, non-sweet pickles, kimchee, sauerkraut, and mustard.

Almost all herbs and spices (no sweeteners and preservatives) and recipe enhancers such as lime juice, lemon, and their grated skins.

Whey protein - keep away from those with sugar, chemical additives, and soy additives

Nuts (make sure there are no sugar-based additives) such as Brazil nuts, hazelnuts, pecans, walnuts, sunflower seeds, sesame and pumpkin seeds, pistachios, pine nuts, and peanuts.

Oils such as coconut oil, pure lard, and olive oil

b. Take the following in moderation

These can be eaten after the initial phase of ketosis has been completed.

Plants:

Bell peppers, shallots, tomatoes - 1 cup has between 10-20 g of carbohydrates and 30-50 calories

Berry varieties, including strawberries, blackberries, cranberries, raspberries, and blueberries. Berries are tricky because while they have an abundance of sugars, they are rich in fiber, which greatly reduces their "net" carbs, or carbohydrates discounted by the fiber they contain.

Cabbage, cauliflower, broccoli, fennel, rutabaga, turnips, Brussels sprouts, and eggplant

Eggplant - 1 cup has 5 g of carbohydrates and 20 calories

Garlic -1 teaspoon has 1 g of carbohydrates and 4 calories

Leeks – The bulbs and lower leaf portions - 1 cup has 15 g of carbohydrates and 50 calories

Mushrooms - 1 cup has 2 g of carbohydrates and 15 calories

Olives - 1 cup has 5 g of carbohydrates and 20 calories

Rhubarb - 1 cup has 5 g of carbohydrates and 20 calories

Onion - 1 cup has 10 g of carbohydrates and 40 calories

Other Peppers- 1 cup has 10 g of carbohydrates and 40 calories

c. Foods that should be avoided at all costs

Alcohol in most forms. Most pure rums and some vodkas though, have zero carbohydrates. Bar beverages and alcohol-based drinks usually have a lot of sugars and syrups and should be avoided.

However, dieters can also consume a variety of beverages in moderation, as long as they contain no sugar. Check the labels carefully on so-called diet sodas to make sure that they do not contain any sugar. Unlimited drinks will include tea, coffee, and heavy cream, minus any refined sugars or sweeteners.

As with most diet plans, water is still the best bet as a beverage alternative. It is a good idea to drink at least half of your body weight in ounces. Plain water can be infused with fresh herbs, such as mint or basil, to provide a little variety. Sodas, flavored waters, sweetened teas, sweetened lemonade, and fruit juices should be avoided.

High-fructose corn-syrup is that deadly stealth sweetener found in most soft drinks, and juices. We mentioned fructose briefly in Chapter 2. If the "high" in high-fructose is not enough to scare someone away, consider that it also functions like a preservative, meaning that not only does it lack B vitamins and other important nutrients, it is chock-full of chemicals that have no business being in the human body.

Avoid grains and sugars in all of their forms. Grains include wheat, barley, rice, rye, sorghum, and anything made from these products. This means that Ketogenic Diet will have no breads, pasta, crackers, and rice. Sugar and anything that contains sugar is also not allowed. This includes white sugar, brown sugar, honey, maple syrup, corn syrup, and brown rice syrup.

There are many names for sugar on the ingredient lists. It's extremely beneficial to familiarize yourself with these names so you will know when a product contains sugar in any form. Be careful of artificial sweeteners like Splenda that could actually be made out of sucralose, which contains carbohydrates.

Breads, including wheat bread

Breakfast cereals

Chocolate bars and candies

Desserts, especially cakes, pies, and pastries

Energy bars, including protein bars

Energy boost drinks - look for sugarless varieties though

Ice cream

Oils that are processed are generally harmful to the body, and will impede Ketogenic progress. These include margarine, sunflower, cottonseed, safflower, canola, grape seed, soybean, and corn oils.

Pancakes and waffles

Rice

Sodas and sugary drinks, including most juice drinks

Syrups and chocolate toppings

T.V. dinners

The basic rule is this: You have to avoid foods and drinks with sugars, carbohydrates, and chemicals.

Chapter 7. Do's and Don'ts

While Ketogenic Diet can provide some awesome benefits, there are many pitfalls to avoid if one is to have success, and even avoid serious hazards to your health.

Mistakes on going on Ketogenic Diet

Because Ketogenic Diet is a radical departure from what most people are used to, it is easy to make mistakes. The following are the most common mistakes that can remove the benefits of Ketogenic Diet, and may even cause harm to your body:

1. To gain the maximum benefits from the diet, you have to be in a state of ketosis for at least two weeks. You CANNOT deviate from this, or you will basically need to start from zero again.

2. Eating too much processed fats and proteins. This is especially true for boxed or T.V. dinners. While they may have a lot of fat content, there are usually a lot of hidden sugars, and worse, artificial chemicals that can derail your progress.

3. Eating more protein as opposed to fat. Fat is the main source of energy, and eating excess protein is bad, because some of it is converted to sugar.

4. Being afraid of fat. In the dietary world, fat is a friend, and we need to forget all the misconceptions about it.

5. Not getting enough water. Sometimes we drink water to accompany carbs, especially sweets, so drastically reducing carbs may cause us to consume less water. Water is the most important element of any diet, and it sometimes helps to give the body a feeling of "fullness."

Chapter 8. Happy Keto Eating Recipes

Meal Plan for Ketogenic Diet

Congratulations! You've gone this far, and now it's time to be rewarded for your persistence and attentiveness.

This chapter will present 7 days' worth of Ketogenic-friendly meals and snacks, which will contain the bare minimum of carbohydrates, while maximizing the consumption of fats and fatty foods. Eating a combination of the meals will guarantee that you will consume less than 50 grams of carbohydrates per day, and should provide a pretty clear picture of the direction that needs to be taken in order to be successful on the diet. Ketogenic Diet requires this proportion in order for the body to achieve ketosis quickly and consistently.

Breakfast Recipes:

1. Ketogenic Breakfast Muffins

Fat Ingredients:

1 medium Egg

1/4 cup Heavy Cream

1 slice cooked Bacon (Cured, Pan-Fried, Cooked)

1 oz. Cheddar Cheese

Other Ingredients:

Salt & Black Pepper (to taste)

How to Prepare:

1. Preheat oven to 350 F.

2. In a bowl, whisk the eggs with the cream and salt and pepper.

3. Spread into pam sprayed muffin tins, and fill the cups 1/2 full.

4. Place 1 slice of crumbled bacon to each muffin and then 1/2 oz. cheese on top of each muffin.

5. Bake for about 15-20 minutes or until slightly browned.

6. Add another 1/2 oz. of cheese onto each muffin and broil until cheese is slightly browned. Enjoy!

2. Ultra Ketogenic Style Egg Breakfast (Serves 2)

Fat Ingredients:

6 organic eggs

½ cup of heavy cream

1 tablespoon of butter

Other Ingredients:

1 cup of shredded spinach

A small pinch Sea Salt+ ground white pepper

1 small onion finely minced

How To Prepare:

1. Take a mixing bowl. Add the eggs, cream, salt and pepper and beat well and put aside.

2. Take a large skillet and heat 1 tablespoon of butter.

3. Then add the onion and spinach and stir constantly.

4. Next, pour the egg mixture and stir until everything becomes scrambled and cooked till light, fluffy and yellow.

5. Serve hot.

3. Bacon & olive omelet (Serves 4)

Fat Ingredients:

8 large free-range eggs

16 thin slices bacon

Other Ingredients:

20 pitted black olives

Pinch of pink Himalayan or sea salt

Freshly ground black pepper

How to Prepare:

1. Cut the olives into thin slices.

2. Lay the bacon, preferably free-range or organic, equally on the surface of the pan and roast for about 5 minutes.

3. Put the eggs into a mixing bowl with a pinch of salt and pepper and beat them well with a whisk or fork.

4. Turn the bacon on the other side when it gets slightly golden in color.

5. Lower the heat and pour in the eggs equally all over the pan.

6. Use a spatula to bring in the omelet from the sides towards the center for the first 30 seconds.

7. Sprinkle with sliced olives and cook for another minute or until the top appears to be almost cooked and firm.

8. Ease the omelet's edges with a spatula. Turn off the heat and serve the omelet on to a plate.

4. Keto Scrambled Eggs (Serves 4)

Fat Ingredients:

8 large eggs

1 tablespoon butter

1 cup shredded Cheddar cheese

½ cup diced sugar-free turkey or chicken ham

¼ cup heavy cream

Other Ingredients:

1 teaspoon salt

½ teaspoon black pepper

½ cup chopped onion

⅓ cup chopped red and green peppers

Chopped scallions for garnish (optional)

How to Prepare:

1. In a large mixing bowl, whisk eggs, cream, salt, and black pepper.

2. Melt the butter in a medium skillet over medium heat. Add egg mixture and stir.

3. When the eggs begin to scramble, add the ham, onion, and peppers.

4. Continue to stir until eggs are almost cooked. Add the cheddar cheese and stir.

5. Flourless Cream Cheese Pancakes (Serves 4)

Fat Ingredients:

4 eggs

4 oz. cream cheese

Other Ingredients:

1 tbsp. cinnamon

2 tbsp. coconut flour

1 packet of Stevia in the Raw

How to Prepare:

1. Combine/mix all the ingredients in a mixing bowl until smooth.

2. Heat up a non-stick pan or skillet on medium high, and coat it with butter or coconut oil.

3. Pour the batter as if it was a regular pancake batter.

4. Cook on one side most of the way before flipping.

5. Top with butter, and/or sugar-free syrup.

6. Keto Eggs Benedict (Serves 4)

Fat Ingredients:

8 large eggs

2 tablespoon butter

8 slices sugar-free Canadian bacon

2 cups Hollandaise Sauce

1 large avocado, cut into 8 pieces

How to Prepare:

1. Heat up a medium skillet over medium-high heat and add the butter. Crack eggs into the pan. Cook for 2 minutes and then flip eggs, using care not to break yolks.

2. Cook for another 2 minutes or until white is completely cooked, but yolk is still runny.

3. Transfer eggs to a plate.

4. Top each egg with a slice of Canadian bacon and a slice of avocado. Pour the sauce onto each egg.

7. High-Fat Ham, Cheese, and Egg Casserole (Serves 6)

Fat Ingredients:

12 large eggs

2 cups cooked diced cooked ham (make sure this does not contain any sugar)

1⁄2 cup shredded mozzarella cheese

1⁄2 cup shredded Cheddar cheese

Other Ingredients:

4 cups broccoli florets

1⁄2 cup chopped scallions

Bunches of broccoli (approximately one cup)

How to Prepare:

1. Preheat oven to 375°F.

2. Fill a large pot with water and bring to a boil. Blanch broccoli by putting in boiling water for 2–3 minutes.

3. Put eggs, ham, mozzarella, cheddar, and scallions in a large bowl and whisk until combined. Add broccoli.

4. Pour into a 9" × 13" baking pan and put in the oven to cook.

Lunch Recipes

1. Stuffed Avocados (Serves 4)

Fat Ingredients:

2 (6-ounce) cans tuna in oil

4 tablespoons mayonnaise

2 large avocados

Other Ingredients:

1 medium green bell pepper, chopped

1 teaspoon dried minced onion

1 teaspoon garlic salt

1 teaspoon black pepper

How to Prepare:

1. Cut avocado in half lengthwise and remove the pit. Set aside.

2. Put tuna, mayonnaise, bell pepper, dried onion, garlic, salt, and black pepper in a medium mixing bowl and mash together with a fork until combined.

3. Scoop half of the mixture into each half of the avocado.

2. Pork Tacos (Serves: 4)

Fat Ingredients:

25 oz. pork mince

½ cup of goat cheese

½ cup of mayonnaise

Other Ingredients:

3 teaspoons Taco Seasoning

4 Romaine Lettuce Leaves

How to Prepare:

1. Place the pork mince in a skillet and cook it for 20 minutes until nice and brown. Leave to cool.

2. Place the pork mince on the lettuce leaves.

3. Add the seasoning, goat cheese and a dollop of mayonnaise.

4. Wrap securely.

3. Chicken Kebabs (Serves up to 5)

Fat Ingredients:

1.5 lbs. chicken tenderloins (approx. 10)

1/2 tbsp. rosemary olive oil (or regular)

Other Ingredients:

10 6" rosemary skewers (soaked in water for at least 1 hour)

A few sprigs of fresh thyme

1/2 tbsp. garlic salt

1/2 tbsp. lemon pepper seasoning

How to Prepare:

1. Preheat oven to 350 degrees.

2. Soak the rosemary skewers for at least 1 hour in water.

3. Use a short sharp knife to twiddle a point on the end of each stick.

4. Toss chicken with ingredients. Slide the leaves off the thyme sprigs and sprinkle them in.

5. Skewer the tenderloin with a rosemary stick.

6. Bake at 350 F for 40 minutes.

4. Sausage Balls (Serves 10 – good to store)

Fat Ingredients:

2 cups of sausages shredded

½ cup of cheddar cheese

½ cup of cottage cheese

1 egg

1 tablespoon butter

Other Ingredients:

1 teaspoon of chili flakes

½ cup of red peppers

¼ teaspoon of mustard powder

How to Prepare:

1. Preheat an oven to 350 degrees.

2. Add the egg, chili, and red peppers in a bowl and mix/whisk until the ingredients are mixed completely.

3. Mix in the remaining ingredients.

4. Using a wooden baking spoon, or cookie scoop, remove the mixture, and hand-roll the sausage into about two dozen sausage balls.

5. Place the formed balls on a buttered baking pan, or cookie sheet.

6. Bake for about 15 minutes. Serve.

7. You may also store the cooked sausage bags in a covered bowl, or sandwich bags in the refrigerator for later use.

5, Tarragon Tuna (Serves 2)

Fat Ingredients:

Two 6-ounce tuna steaks, 1 inch thick

2 teaspoons mayonnaise

1 teaspoon olive oil

Other Ingredients:

2 tablespoons minced fresh or 2 teaspoons dried tarragon plus tarragon sprigs for garnish

Salt and cracked pepper to taste

How to Prepare:

1. Stir together the mayo and tarragon in a small bowl. Cover and set aside.

2. Heat a heavy skillet or ridged grill pan over medium-high heat.

3. Pat the tuna dry with paper towels, then season to taste with salt and cracked pepper. Dab olive oil over the surfaces of the fish.

4. Pan grilled the fish for about 3 minutes per side for medium. Transfer to warmed dinner plates.

5. Top each steak with a dollop of tarragon mayonnaise, and garnish with tarragon sprigs. Place a mound of squash beside the tuna.

6. Tuna and Egg Salad (Serves 2)

Fat Ingredients:

2 large hard-boiled eggs

2 (6-ounce) cans tuna (try to get those packed in oil

½ cup mayonnaise

Other Ingredients:

¼ cup diced white onion

¼ cup sugar-free relish

½ teaspoon salt

½ teaspoon black pepper

How to Prepare:

1. Put eggs in a medium mixing bowl and mash with a fork. Add tuna and mayonnaise and mash together until ingredients are combined.

2. Stir in onion, relish, salt, and pepper.

7. Chicken Avocado Salad (Serves 2)

Fat Ingredients:

1 (12.5-ounce) can shredded chicken breast

½ cup Homemade Mayonnaise

1 teaspoon olive oil

1 medium avocado, cubed

Other Ingredients:

2 tablespoons sliced black olives

½ teaspoon garlic salt

½ teaspoon black pepper

¼ teaspoon paprika

1 teaspoon fresh lemon juice

How to Prepare:

Put all ingredients in a medium mixing bowl and mash with a fork until combined.

Dinner Recipes

1. Carb-less Pork Skewers (Serves 4)

<u>Fat Ingredients:</u>

2 lbs. pork shoulder

1 cup virgin olive oil (may be reused later on)

<u>Other ingredients:</u>

Juice from 2 large lemons

2 tbsp. balsamic vinegar

4 tbsp. freshly chopped mint

4 tbsp. freshly chopped oregano

2 tsp. sea salt

Dash of freshly ground black pepper

4 wooden or stainless steel skewers

<u>How to Prepare:</u>

1. To prepare the marinade, rinse the mint and oregano and drain thoroughly. Chop the herbs and preserve these apart in a small bowl.

2. Cube the pork into big cubes. Place them in a medium bowl and pour the olive oil on them.

3. Add the chopped herbs and season with balsamic vinegar. Season with salt and freshly grounded black pepper to taste.

4. Combine all the ingredients, and ensure the meat is submerged in oil. Let it relax in the fridge for 8 to 12 hours.

5. When the meat is marinated, use the grill to preheat the oven to 450 degrees. Note that the meat will barely change color after you take it out from the fridge. This is fine.

6. Skewer the meat pieces in four skewer sticks. Place them on a rack and within the oven.

7. After about 10 minutes, flip the skewers, and cook until done.

2. Sea Bass with Mango Chutney, Ginger, and Black Sesame Seeds (Makes 2 servings)

Fat Ingredients:

Two 6-ounce striped bass fillets

1 tablespoon sesame oil

Cooking spray

Other Ingredients:

1 tablespoon minced fresh ginger (see note)

1 tablespoon soy sauce

Salt and freshly milled black pepper to taste

¼ cup mango chutney

3 cups shredded iceberg lettuce

Ginger and Hot Red Pepper Vinaigrette

How to Prepare:

1. Preheat the oven to 425°F. Spray an 8 X 8 X 8-inch Pyrex baking dish with cooking spray.

2. Place the fillets in the baking dish. Sprinkle each fillet with ginger, soy sauce, and sesame oil. Lightly salt and pepper. Cover the dish with foil and bake for 10 minutes.

3. Remove from the oven and spoon 2 tablespoons of chutney onto each fillet. Return to the oven and bake, uncovered, for 5 more minutes.

4. Toss the shredded lettuce with the dressing. Divide between two plates and top each one with a fillet.

3. Roasted Butterfish (Serves 4)

Fat Ingredients:

Four giant butterfish fillets

8 tablespoon butter or ghee

Other Ingredients:

4 cloves garlic

4 teaspoons freshly chopped thyme

Pinch sea salt

Juice from 1 lemon

How to Prepare:

1. Begin by seasoning the butterfish fillets with a little bit of salt and place them on a plate.

2. Soften the butter, add the herbs and crushed garlic and blend all the pieces collectively in a small bowl.

3. Pour the butter combination over the fish.

4. Warm a non-stick pan over medium heat and add the fish.

5. Roast for about 2 to 3 minutes on both sides until cooked and the fish will get a crispy golden texture. Be certain that the fillet is totally cooked by slicing into it. Cooked flesh will look opaque.

6. Place the fish onto a serving plate and squeeze a little bit of lemon over it. Serve sizzling.

4. Broccoli and Ham Quiche (Serves 12)

Fat Ingredients:

10 large organic eggs or 12 medium eggs

2 cups of thinly sliced ham

1 cup of grated cheddar cheese

1 ½ cups of heavy cream

3 tablespoons of olive oil

Other Ingredients:

12 cups of cubed broccoli flowerets

2 teaspoons of chili flakes

How to Prepare:

1. Preheat the oven to 350F.

2. Take 2 deep 10-inch quiche pans. Grease them with a bit of olive oil and keep aside.

3. Take a large mixing bowl. Crack all the eggs and pour into the bowl. Then add the heavy cream, chili flakes, and beat well until it has all been mixed well.

4. Take each quiche pan and place the ham slices and broccoli flowerets evenly in each pan. Then sprinkle the cheese over them and finally pour the egg and cream mixture over it.

5. Bake for 20 minutes until the top is golden brown in color. Prick with a fork till the bottom of quiche to check if done. If it is clean, then the quiche is ready to enjoy.

5. Baked Salmon (Serves 4)

Fat Ingredients:

4 6-ounce salmon fillets

3 tbsp. olive oil

Other Ingredients:

2 tablespoons of lemon juice

1 tablespoon each of minced parsley, mint, garlic, paprika, sunflower seeds (slightly crushed)

How to Prepare:

1. Clean the fillet and put aside.

2. Place all the other ingredients in another bowl, and mix well and pour onto the fish. Marinate the fillet for 6 hours.

3. After 6 hours, place in a baking dish and bake for 1 hour at 250F until flaky and cooked.

4. Serve with sour cream, green beans and apricots.

6. Fried Chicken (Serves 4)

<u>Fat Ingredients:</u>

1 pound or 4 (4-ounce) boneless, skinless chicken breasts

1/2 cup crushed pork rinds

1/2 cup grated Parmesan cheese

2 large eggs

2 tablespoons coconut oil

<u>Other Ingredients:</u>

1/2 teaspoon garlic powder

1/4 teaspoon onion powder

1/4 teaspoon dried minced onion

1/4 teaspoon salt

1/4 teaspoon black pepper

<u>How to Prepare:</u>

1. Put pork rinds, Parmesan cheese, garlic powder, onion powder, minced onion, salt, and black pepper in a large mixing bowl and stir until well mixed.

2. Crack eggs into a separate bowl and whisk.

3. Dip each chicken breast into eggs and then coat in pork rind mixture, making sure the chicken is completely covered.

4. Heat coconut oil in a skillet over medium-high heat. Place the chicken breasts into the pan. Let them cook for 5–7 minutes or until pork rind crust is browned. Flip chicken over and let them cook for another 5–7 minutes until cooked through.

5. Serve hot.

7. One Pan Baked Chicken Thighs (Serves 2)

Fat Ingredients:

4 chicken thighs (deboned, skin on)

1/4 cup olive oil

Other Ingredients:

2 zucchinis

1/2 cup carrot (sliced)

2 tablespoons balsamic vinegar

1 cup daikon radish

1-inch length of cube ginger, minced

How to Prepare:

1. Pre-heat an oven to 350 degrees.

2. Use a paper towel, and pat the chicken thighs dry.

3. Wrap the skins around the chicken thighs, and place these on a buttered or greased baking sheet.

4. Slice the radish and zucchinis, and with the carrots, place them around the thigh pieces.

5. Using a small bowl mix the vinegar, oil, and ginger – this is your sauce. Pour the mix over the chicken.

5. Season with salt and pepper and bake the chicken thighs for 30 minutes.

<u>Conclusion</u>

I hope this book was able to help you to achieve not only your weight loss goals, but to have a more vibrant, healthier lifestyle beyond losing weight and looking great.

The next step in your journey is to start listing down your weight goals, changing your food shopping lists, and prepare for a new and sexier wardrobe!

Finally, if you enjoyed this book, then I'd like to ask you for a

favor, would you be kind enough to leave a review for this book on Amazon? It'd be greatly appreciated!

Thank you and good luck!

REFERENCES

Introduction

1. Brown, H. (2015). Planning to Go on a Diet? One Word of Advice: Don't. Retrieved December 30, 2016, from http://www.slate.com/articles/health_and_science/medical_examiner/2015/03/diets_do_not_work_the_thin_evidence_that_losing_weight_makes_you_healthier.html

2. Average woman spends 31 years on a diet, researchers say. (2007). Retrieved December 30, 2016, from http://www.dailymail.co.uk/health/article-430913/Average-woman-spends-31-years-diet-researchers-say.html

Chapter 1. The False Promises of Carbohydrates

1. Office of Dietary Supplements - Daily Values (DVs). (n.d.). Retrieved December 18, 2016, from https://ods.od.nih.gov/HealthInformation/dailyvalues.aspx
2. USDA "Plate"

2. Choose MyPlate. (n.d.). Retrieved December 25, 2016, from https://www.choosemyplate.gov/

3. Longevity/Health in Ancient Paleolithic vs Neolithic Peoples. (n.d.). Retrieved December 20, 2016, from http://www.beyondveg.com/nicholson-w/angel-1984/angel-1984-1a.shtml

4. DeWitte, S. N., & Bekvalac, J. (2010). Oral Health and Frailty in the Medieval English Cemetery of St. Mary Graces. Retrieved December 22, 2016, from https://www.ncbi.nlm.nih.gov/pmc/articles/PMC3094918/

5. A Brief History of Heart Disease. (n.d.). Retrieved December 22, 2016, from http://forum.prisonplanet.com/index.php?topic=206436.0

Chapter 2. The Chemistry of Eating

1. McDonald, L., & McDonald, L. (1998). The ketogenic diet: a complete guide for the dieter and practitioner. Austin, TX: The Author.

2. Metabolic processes (2010). Retrieved December 26, 2016, from https://www.youtube.com/watch?v=mtHDjC1emGs

3. Overview Metabolism. (n.d.). Retrieved December 24, 2016, from http://chemistry.elmhurst.edu/vchembook/600glycolysis.html

Chapter 3. How We Get Fat And Sick From Food

1. Cordain, L. (2011). The Paleo diet: lose weight and get healthy by eating the foods you were designed to eat. Hoboken, NJ: Wiley.

Chapter 4. Ketosis And Ketogenesis

1. Boyers, Lindsay (2015). The everything guide to the ketogenic diet: a step-by-step guide to the ultimate fat-burning diet plan! Avon, MA: Adams Media.

2. Ray, N. (2013). Atkins diet: complete Atkins diet guide to losing weight and feeling amazing! North Charleston, SC: Createspace.

Chapter 5. Ketogenic Diet Basics

1. Excellent carb-counting resource include:

http://www.carb-counter.net/

2. There are a great multitude of apps for both Android and IOS. Listed below is a tiny sample of what's available:

Calorie, Carb & Fat Counter by Virtuagym

Calorie Counter by My Fitness Pal

Low Carb Foods Guide by deluxapps

3. Boyers, Lindsay (2015). The everything guide to the ketogenic diet: a step-by-step guide to the ultimate fat-burning diet plan! Avon, MA: Adams Media.

4. (2016). Retrieved December 26, 2016, from https://www.youtube.com/watch?v=H7mjm9LyW-c

Chapter 6. What to Eat. And What Not To!

1. H. (2016). Complete Keto Diet Food List: What to Eat and Avoid | The KetoDiet Blog. Retrieved December 24, 2016, from http://ketodietapp.com/Blog/post/2015/01/03/Keto-Diet-Food-List-What-to-Eat-and-Avoid

2, Johnson, R. A., Says, R., Says, J. R., Says, C., Says, L., Says, L., . . . Says, A. (2016). The Ultimate Ketogenic Diet Food List (What to Eat on The Keto Diet). Retrieved December 22, 2016, from https://dietingwell.com/ketogenic-diet-food-list/

3. H. (2016). Ketogenic Diet Food List - What Are Keto Foods? (PDF Download). Retrieved December 20, 2016, from http://paleomagazine.com/ketogenic-diet-food-list

Chapter 7. Do's and Don't's

1. H. (2016). How To Low Carb: 15 Common Weight Loss Mistakes | The KetoDiet Blog. Retrieved December 27, 2016, from http://ketodietapp.com/Blog/post/2016/01/11/how-to-low-carb-15-common-weight-loss-mistakes

2. 13 common keto mistakes. (2016). Retrieved December 22, 2016, from https://www.ketovangelist.com/13-common-keto-mistakes/

Chapter 8. Happy Keto Eating Recipes

1. Slajerova, M. (2016). Sweet & savory fat bombs: 100 delicious treats for fat fasts, ketogenic, paleo, and low-carb diets. Beverly, MA: Fair Winds.

2. The Best Keto Recipes. (n.d.). Retrieved December 23, 2016, from https://www.dietdoctor.com/low-carb/recipes/best-keto-recipes

3. Low Carb Recipes for Ketogenic Diets. (n.d.). Retrieved December 27, 2016, from http://www.ketogenic-diet-resource.com/low-carb-recipes.html

Other Titles by Steve Blum

Atkins Diet: Break Out from the Fat Prison for Good

Intermittent Fasting: Lose up to 1 Pound a Day, Get a Beautiful Lean Body and Master Your Hunger

Ketosis Diet: 30 Day Plan for Optimal, Super-Effective Fat Loss with Ketogenic Diet